The Little Library of Healing Herbs

Meditatives

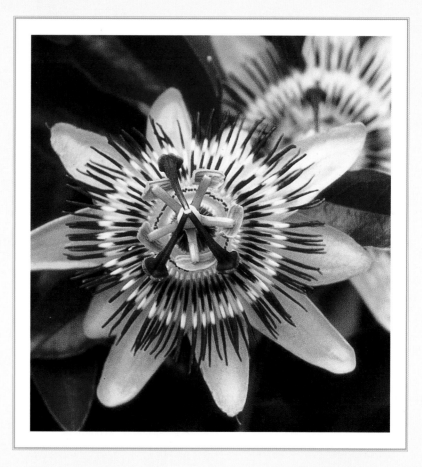

The Little Library of Healing Herbs

Meditatives

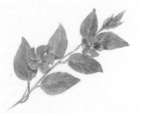

PAST TIMES

PAST TIMES®

www.past-times.com

This edition published by PAST TIMES in 2004

01 03 05 04 02
1 3 5 7 9 10 8 6 4 2

The Little Library of Healing Herbs was created and produced by
Carroll & Brown Publishers Limited
20 Lonsdale Road London NW6 6RD

Written and compiled by Ian Wood
Copyright © Carroll & Brown Limited 2004

A CIP catalogue record for this book is available from the British Library.

ISBN 1-903258-99-5

Reproduced by RDC, Malaysia

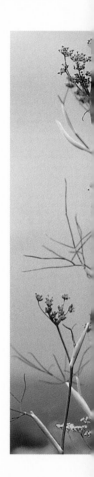

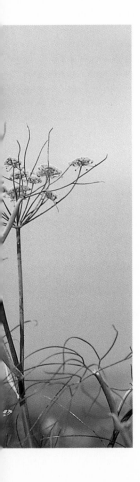

CONTENTS

INTRODUCTION

Please note that although herbs are natural products and most are safe to use, in some circumstances they can have harmful effects. If you have any allergies or other medical conditions, if you are pregnant or breastfeeding, or if you are taking any form of medication (including oral contraceptives), consult your doctor or a herbalist before using any herbal remedy.

MANY HERBS HAVE THE POWER to calm and soothe the mind, helping to relieve stress and anxiety and enhancing our emotional and spiritual lives. You can use their colours and aromas simply to create a peaceful atmosphere in your home, or to help you to meditate and achieve inner peace and serenity.

Meditation is easy to learn and has many benefits for both mind and body. Scientific studies have shown that regular meditation relieves stress, anxiety, depression, and insomnia, and makes you calmer and happier. It also gives a helpful boost to many of your body's essential systems, including those that are often harmed by stress – regular meditation will improve the functions of your immune and digestive systems, and by reducing your heart rate and lowering your blood pressure it will make you less likely to suffer a heart attack or a stroke.

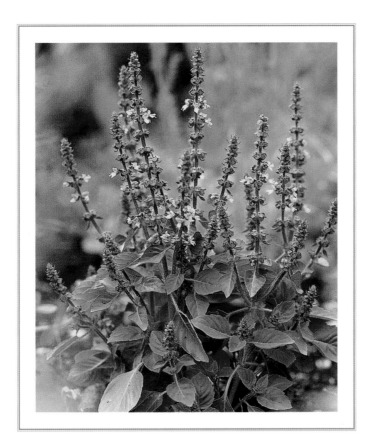

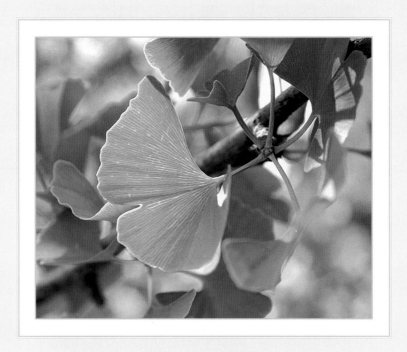

"This leaf from a tree in the East,
Has been given to my garden.
It reveals a certain secret,
Which pleases me and thoughtful people."

Johann Wolfgang von Goethe
Ginkgo biloba
1815

Preparing for Meditation

WHEN YOU WANT TO MEDITATE, or simply relax to unwind and rid yourself of stress, first spend a little time creating a peaceful environment free from unwanted distractions. You don't need to make any elaborate preparations – all you need is a clean, comfortable, and quiet space that will allow you forget the outside world and let your mind become still.

Tidy your room, close the door, and draw the curtains or blinds; close the windows, too, if noises from outside are likely to intrude on your tranquillity. For lighting, use a small table lamp instead of the ceiling light, or illuminate the room with the gentle, calming flicker of candles. Make sure the room is reasonably warm, because your body temperature will drop as you relax, and switch off or unplug your phone to avoid being disturbed by incoming calls.

THE HERBAL CABINET

Potpourris

By preparing your own potpourris you can create an aromatic haven, using the herbs, spices, and scented flowers that you find most appealing. Calming and soothing or invigorating and restorative, potpourris can change the mood in any room and make it easier for you to focus your mind for your forthcoming meditation.

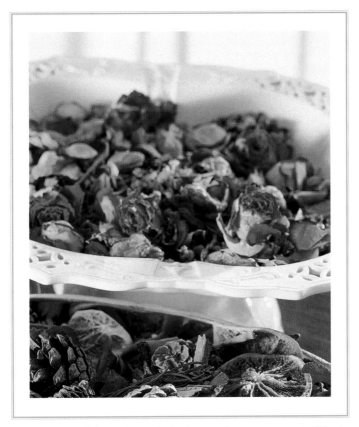

Experiment with your favourite herbs to make your own special blend.

Simple Meditation

THERE ARE MANY DIFFERENT MEDITATION TECHNIQUES, but meditating is really about "being" rather than doing, and all you need is a quiet space and about half an hour of your time. To begin, sit or lie in a comfortable position, close your eyes, and breathe deeply and slowly through your nose with your mouth closed. Next, consciously relax the muscles in each part of your body, starting at your toes and working up to your neck and head.

When your body is completely relaxed, let your cares and worries leave your mind, and concentrate on your breathing. If thoughts enter your mind, let them float out again when you exhale. Enjoy this meditative state for as long as you wish, then open your eyes and sit or lie quietly for a few minutes to allow it to fade gently away as your mind returns to its normal conscious state.

THE HERBAL CABINET

Some of the best herbs for meditation include lavender, clary sage, and rosemary. The floral-herby scent of lavender is soothing and balancing and will aid you in freeing your mind of everyday cares. Clary sage also has calming qualities, and its nutty aroma is said to produce a mild feeling of intoxication and encourage creative thinking. The distinctive piney smell of rosemary will make your meditation refreshing and invigorating.

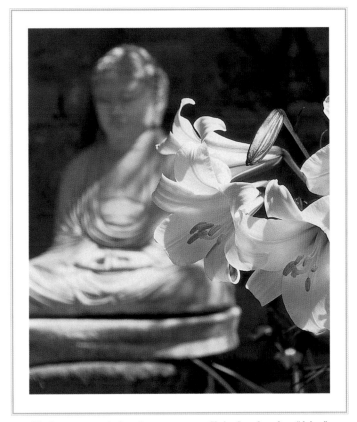

Unclutter your mind and concentrate on "being" rather than "doing".

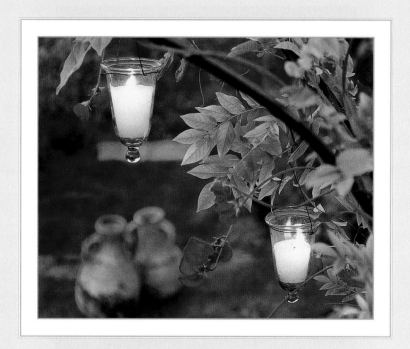

"He that in his studies wholly applies himself
to labour and exercise, and neglects
meditation, loses his time ..."

CONFUCIUS
c. 479 BC

Symbolic Herbs

In pre-Christian northern Europe, the cowslip was associated with Freya, goddess of love, and it represented the keys to Freya's treasure. When Christian lore supplanted these pagan beliefs, the Virgin Mary replaced Freya, and Freya's keys became St Peter's keys to the gates of heaven.

FOR THOUSANDS OF YEARS, people have invested certain herbs and flowers with religious or magical significance. They have used these plants as symbols of particular gods, goddesses, or saints, and to represent or invoke qualities such as love, luck, and happiness.

In India, for example, holy basil is offered in reverence to the Hindu gods Vishnu and Krishna, but many cultures associate it with love and the Haitians use sweet basil as an offering to Erzulie, the voodoo goddess of love. In the West, the Madonna lily symbolizes the Virgin Mary and is said to confer protection from harm, and the passionflower represents the suffering of Christ and brings peace and friendship. Marigold is believed to promote prophetic dreams and psychic powers, while the humble cowslip (*Primula veris*) is associated with healing and happiness and with the Virgin Mary and St Peter.

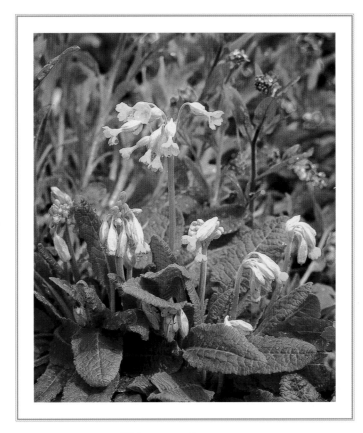

Primula veris

Calming Colours

In Egyptian mythology, the art of healing with colours was given to us by Thoth, the ibis-headed lord of the Moon, lord of time, and god of learning and writing. Thoth entered Greek mythology as Hermes Trismegistus (Hermes the thrice-greatest), the god of wisdom and learning who vanquished Typhon, the dragon of ignorance.

THE EFFECTS THAT DIFFERENT COLOURS can have on the mind has been known since ancient times, and the Egyptians and Greeks used coloured minerals, stones, and crystals in therapies designed to cure mental and physical ailments. They used shades of red, orange, and yellow to stimulate; blues, indigos, and violets to calm and rejuvenate; and white to strengthen.

Sprigs of blue-, purple-, or white-flowering herbs placed in your meditation room will enhance your clarity of mind, balance your emotions, and promote a meditative state of mind. Blue is traditionally the colour of meditation and spiritual expansion, purple is purifying, and white promotes spirituality. The effect of the coloured herbs will be enhanced if you choose those that are also calming by nature, such as lavender, skullcap (*Scutellaria spp.*), clary sage, or valerian.

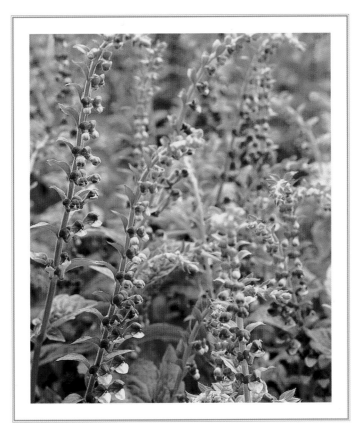

Scutellaria spp.

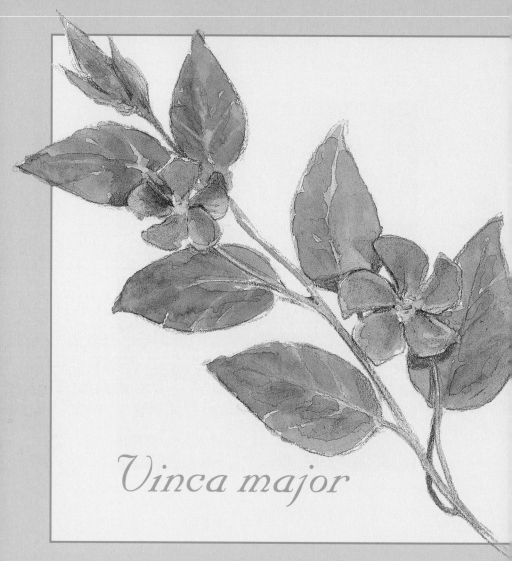

Vinca major

Periwinkle

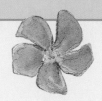

*T*he periwinkles are attractive perennial shrubs with glossy, dark green leaves, sometimes streaked with lighter green, and flowers that can be blue, purple, crimson, pink, or white. In the past, periwinkles were known as "sorcerer's violets" because they were associated with magic and spells, and were thought to have the power to drive away evil spirits and witches – no witch would enter a house that had periwinkles growing at the door. Periwinkles also symbolized happy memories and had a reputation for promoting thoughts of love.

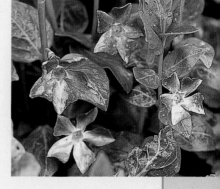

The most common species are the greater periwinkle (*Vinca major*), the lesser periwinkle (*Vinca minor*), and the Madagascar periwinkle (*Vinca rosea*). These are grown mainly as decorative plants, but their leaves and flowers (especially those of the lesser periwinkle) also have uses in herbal medicine, for instance in remedies for headaches, vertigo, and memory problems.

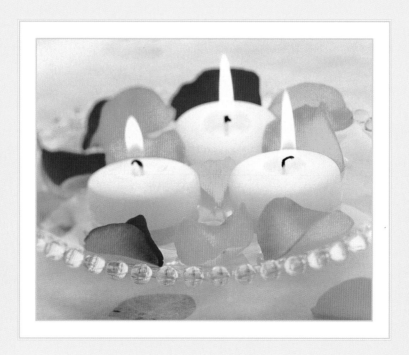

"Colours seen by candle-light
Will not look the same by day."

ELIZABETH BARRETT BROWNING
THE LADY'S YES
1844

Calm the Spirit

MEDITATION IS A GREAT WAY TO RELIEVE STRESS or nervousness, but sometimes these unsettling feelings can make it hard to clear your mind of troubling thoughts and achieve a state of meditative calm. When this happens, you may find it helpful to try a gentle herbal nerve tonic that will soothe both mind and spirit.

Vervain (*verbena officinalis*), cowslip, and gingko, made into teas, are all herbs with a proven record for easing troubled minds. Vervain is a traditional remedy for anxiety, exhaustion, and depression, and cowslip eases anxiety, irritability, and nervous excitability. Ginkgo improves blood circulation throughout the body and especially in the brain, making it an effective mood improver that also boosts mental alertness and memory. It is said to be particularly beneficial for older people.

THE HERBAL CABINET

Herbal Teas

To make vervain, ginkgo, or cowslip tea, put 2 tablespoonfuls of fresh (or 1 tablespoonful of dried) vervain or ginkgo leaves, or 2 tablespoonfuls of fresh cowslip petals, into a cup. Fill it with boiling water, leave it to steep for 5 to 10 minutes, then strain out the leaves or petals and drink it. For best effect, drink two or three cups a day.

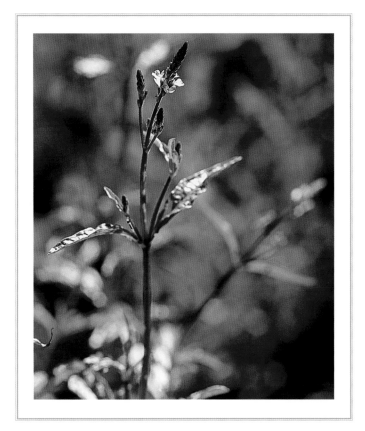

Verbena

Ginkgo

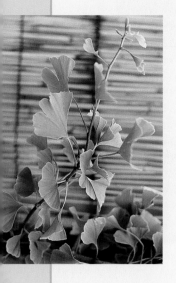

The ginkgo tree is the sole survivor of an ancient order of plants, the Ginkgoales, that date back more than 270 million years and were around when dinosaurs roamed the Earth. Today, in its native habitat of central China, the ginkgo grows with one or more main trunks and spreading branches, and can reach a height of 40 m (130 feet). The ginkgo was introduced into Europe in the late seventeenth century by German botanist Engelbert Kaempfer (1651–1716), who brought seeds from Japan to the botanical garden in Utrecht, Holland, where one of the trees grown from his seeds still stands.

Highly regarded in traditional Chinese and Japanese medicine, and used for treating disorders of the heart, lungs, and urinary system, in the West, ginkgo is a popular herbal medicine because of its ability to improve memory and other mental functions.

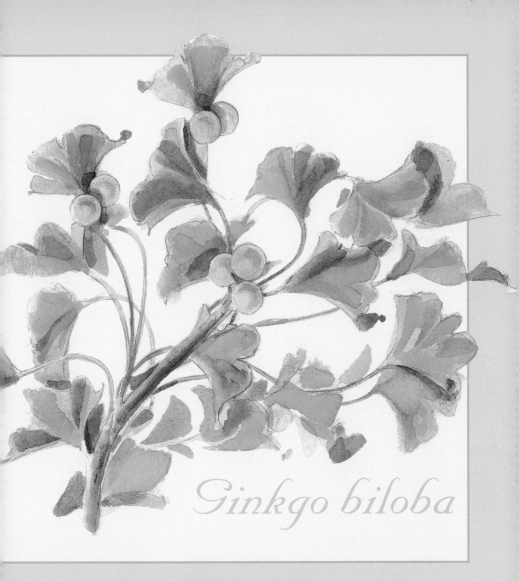

Ginkgo biloba

Calming Aromas

THE SWEET, EVOCATIVE AROMAS OF FRAGRANT HERBS will calm the spirit and clear the mind, so they have long been used to aid and enhance meditation and religious devotions. The aromas can come from sprigs or garlands of fresh herbs, from herb oils, from herb-scented candles, or from dried herbs sprinkled into a bowl of hot water, onto glowing charcoal, or burned as incense.

The many varieties of basil have strong, uplifting scents. Holy basil, for example, has a clove-like aroma and is greatly valued as an aid to meditation in India, where it is frequently planted around Hindu shrines and rosaries made from its cut stems are used as meditation beads. Calming, refreshing lavender soothes the mind and body, balances the emotions, and increases mental alertness, while thyme and rosemary will help to clear the mind and improve memory and concentration.

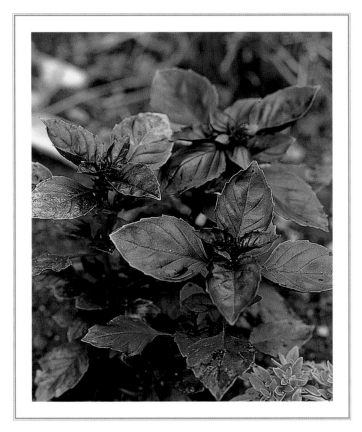

Ocimum

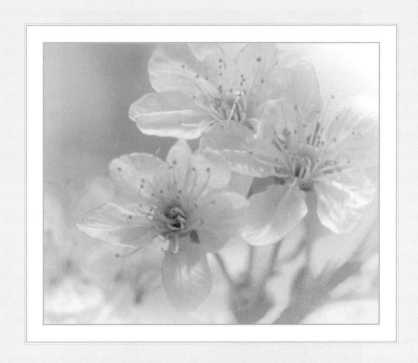

"Some happy tone
Of meditation, slipping in between
The beauty coming and the beauty gone."

WILLIAM WORDSWORTH
MOST SWEET IT IS
1835

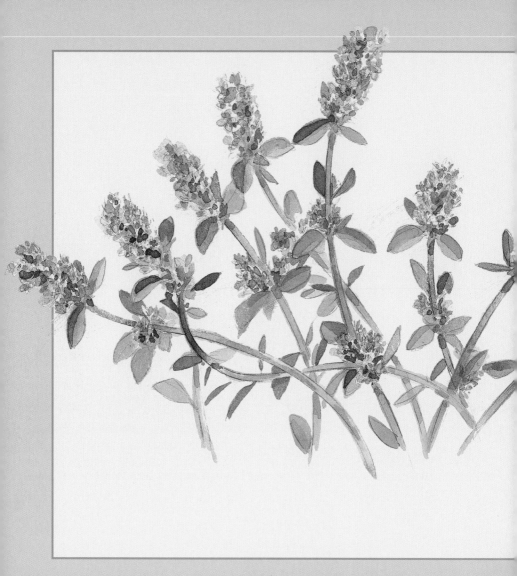

Thyme

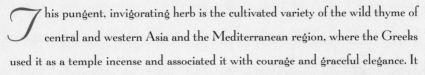

This pungent, invigorating herb is the cultivated variety of the wild thyme of central and western Asia and the Mediterranean region, where the Greeks used it as a temple incense and associated it with courage and graceful elegance. It has long been a popular culinary herb, and people used to plant it near beehives because the insects loved feeding on it and its nectar improved the flavour of their honey. Thyme is also an important medicinal herb, because its main active ingredient, thymol, is a powerful antiseptic and an effective mouthwash and cough remedy.

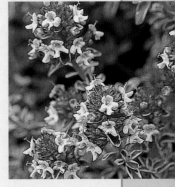

Thyme is a small perennial shrub that usually reaches a height of no more than 10 to 20 cm (4 to 8 inches) and grows best in well-drained, lime-rich soil. Its paired leaves are small and greenish-grey in colour, and its pale, purple-white flowers are in bloom throughout the summer months.

Scented Bath Oils and Candles

BATHING IS AN IMPORTANT SOURCE OF MEDITATIVE RELAXATION, and oils and bath salts scented with soothing herbs such as lavender, rosemary, or thyme will create an atmosphere of tranquillity that promotes calm and mental clarity. An aromatic bath can undoubtedly benefit your health and well-being, with the vapours from the scented oil or salts being inhaled as you relax and unwind.

When a herb-scented candle burns, the heat of the melting wax releases the fragrance of the herbs so that it diffuses around the room. Dip an unscented candle into melted candle wax then roll it in finely powdered dried herbs. Alternatively, you could buy a candle-making kit and mix pure herb oil into the wax when you make the candles. Add about 10 drops of herb oil to each half-kilo (pound) of melted wax, and stir well to blend the oil in evenly.

THE HERBAL CABINET

The bathroom is often overlooked as a place of relaxation and refuge, but there are several things you can do to increase its meditative ambience. Place some plants in your bathroom to promote the circulation of chi energy; ensure your bathroom colours are harmonious – blue and green, the colours of healing and beauty, are especially suitable for the bathroom.

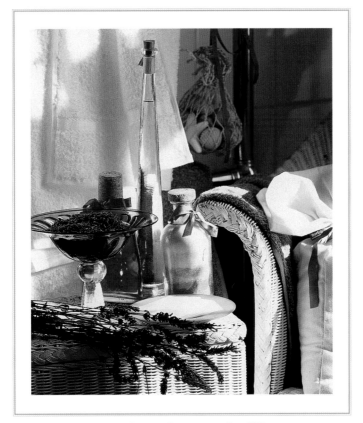

Make your bathroom a haven away from life's stresses.

Incense for Meditation

The use of incense probably dates back to prehistoric times, because it was mentioned in some of the earliest surviving works of literature. These include the Sumerian text of the Epic of Gilgamesh, the story of King Gilgamesh of Uruk in what is now southern Iraq. The text was written down about 2,700 years ago but based on a story dating back to at least a thousand years earlier.

FOR THOUSANDS OF YEARS, people have used the scented smoke of burning incense to create a mystical, spiritual environment for meditation and prayer. Incense is made from a variety of aromatic ingredients, including resins, gums, oils, and herbs, which are blended together and formed into sticks or cones or used loose as small balls, granules, or powders. Solid incenses are burned in holders that support them safely and catch any hot ash that drops from them, and loose incenses are usually sprinkled onto hot charcoal inside a small brass pot.

Herbal incenses for home use are easy to make and a pleasure to use. A blend of lavender, rosemary, and vetiver, for example, will create a fragrance that calms the mind and balances the emotions, while a mix of lavender, rosemary, and peppermint produces a comforting aroma that promotes a sense of inner warmth.

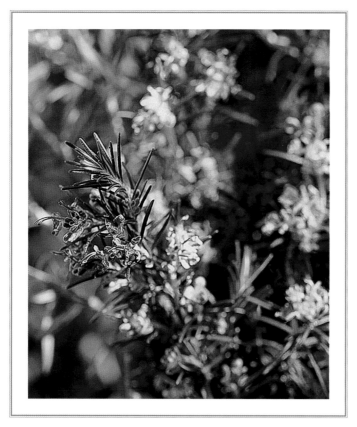

Rosmarinus officinalis

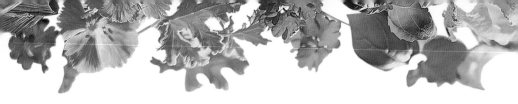

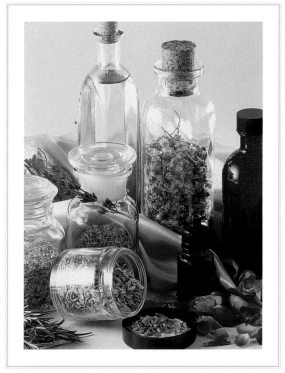

Use your dried herbs and herb oils to create your own incense recipes for a very personal meditation.

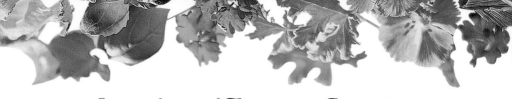

Lavender and Rosemary Incense

2 tbsp rose petals
2 tbsp lavender flowers
1 tbsp rosemary leaves
1 tsp powdered vetiver
$^1/_2$ tsp oil of lavender
$^1/_2$ tsp oil of rosemary
2 tsp orrisroot powder

Grind the flowers and rosemary together in a mortar and pestle and combine with the rest of the ingredients in a bowl. Store the mixture in a dark, airtight container for 2–3 months to allow it to mature, then use it by sprinkling a little on burning charcoal or on the fire.

Honeyed Herb Incense

The comforting fragrance released by this sweet incense releases your mind from the cares of the day, in readiness for your meditation.

4 tsp honey
4 tbsp water
1 tbsp lavender flowers
1 tbsp rosemary leaves
1 tbsp peppermint leaves

Combine the honey and water, then mix the herbs together and gradually rub the honey and water into them. Leave to macerate in a bowl for 2–3 days, stirring regularly, until the mixture is drying but not completely dry, and still sticky. Then take small amounts of the mixture, roll them into small balls, and store them in an airtight container. To burn them, place them safely on a heatproof surface and light until they begin to smoulder and smoke.

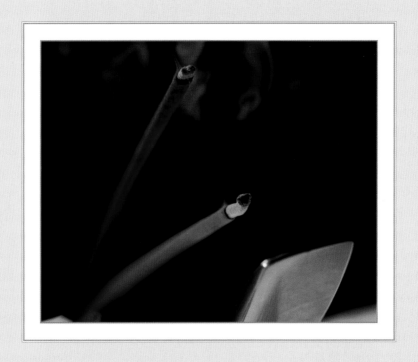

"O blest unfabled Incense Tree
That burns in glorious Araby
With red scent chalicing the air,
Till earth-life grow Elysian there!"

GEORGE DARLEY
NEPENTHE
1835

Smudging

In Native American tradition, smudging is important in ceremonies and rituals and has many uses including banishing negative energies, attracting positive energies and loving spirits, and purifying and promoting psychic awareness. Herbs used for smudging include white sage (Salvia apiana), desert sage (Artemesia tridentata), and mugwort (Artemesia vulgaris).

AS AN ALTERNATIVE TO USING INCENSE, you can burn sprigs or wands of dried aromatic herbs so that their smoke creates a cleansing, calming atmosphere for meditation. Good herbs to use include sage, clary sage, lavender, rosemary, basil, peppermint, and thyme. The traditional Native American version of this is known as "smudging", a ritual act of burning bundles of herbs (called smudge sticks) for ceremonial inner cleansing and for initiating religious ceremonies.

To burn sprigs of herbs, put them in a heatproof bowl and light them, then blow out the flames and allow the sprigs to smoulder and smoke. To use a wand or smudge stick, hold one end over a lighted candle until the tip begins to smoulder. Then blow out the flames and waft the smoking stick around the room or put it safely in a heatproof bowl where it can smoulder gently away.

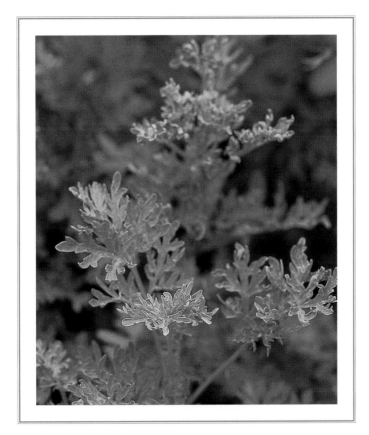

Artemesia

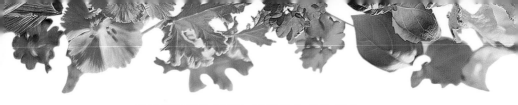

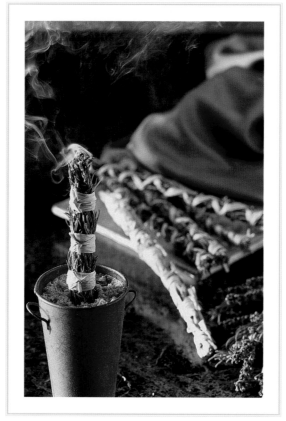

Herbal Wands and Smudge Sticks

When lit, these highly evocative aromatic wands intensify the
heady scents of your chosen herbs.

**Choose from:
lavender, rosemary,
sage, clary sage,
basil, peppermint,
thyme**

To make herbal wands, hold a few fresh herb sprigs
together and tie them tightly at one end with thread or
(preferably) raffia. Hang the bundles up until the herbs
have almost but not completely dried, then bind the
entire length of each bundle with thread or raffia in a
criss-cross pattern.

To make smudge sticks, use bigger bundles of herbs
and bind just the lower halves instead of the entire
lengths of the herbs.

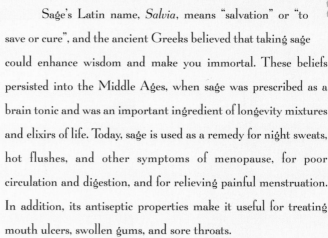

Sage

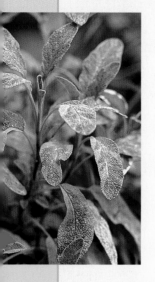

S age, also called garden sage or common sage, is an evergreen shrub that grows to around 30 cm (one foot) or more high and has hairy, greyish-green leaves and purplish flowers. Originally native to the Mediterranean countries, it is now grown widely as a culinary and medicinal herb all over the world.

Sage's Latin name, *Salvia*, means "salvation" or "to save or cure", and the ancient Greeks believed that taking sage could enhance wisdom and make you immortal. These beliefs persisted into the Middle Ages, when sage was prescribed as a brain tonic and was an important ingredient of longevity mixtures and elixirs of life. Today, sage is used as a remedy for night sweats, hot flushes, and other symptoms of menopause, for poor circulation and digestion, and for relieving painful menstruation. In addition, its antiseptic properties make it useful for treating mouth ulcers, swollen gums, and sore throats.

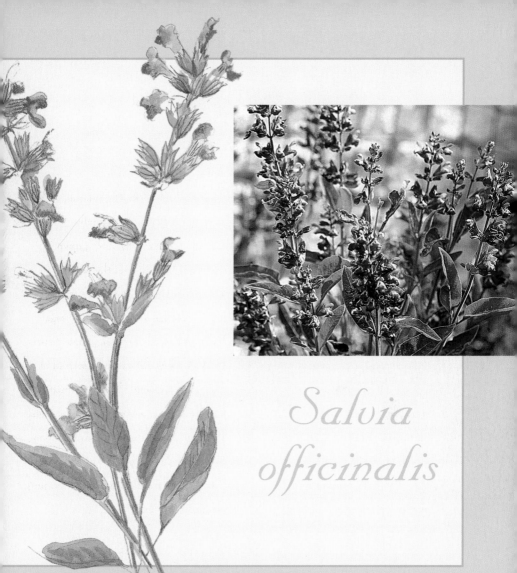

Salvia
officinalis

The Language of Herbs

LIKE FLOWERS, DIFFERENT HERBS have come to be associated with different thoughts, emotions, and qualities. Usually, these associations are quite straightforward – bergamot, for example, signifies compassion, and periwinkle represents love and sweet memories – but sometimes they are contradictory, so basil symbolizes both love and hatred, and calendula embodies both joy and grief.

Basil best wishes, love, hatred

Bay leaf strength, glory

Bergamot compassion

Borage courage, bluntness, talent

Burdock tenacity

Calendula joy, envy, grief

Chamomile humility, patience

Chervil sincerity

Coriander lust, hidden worth

Cowslip pensiveness, healing

Dandelion faithfulness, happiness, love's oracle

Eucalyptus protection

Fennel praiseworthiness, strength

Feverfew protection

Garlic courage, strength

Hyssop cleanliness, wards away evil spirits

Jasmine sensuality, wealth, elegance

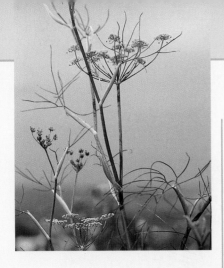

Juniper succour, protection

Lavender devotion, distrust

Lemon Balm sympathy, brings love

Lemon Verbena unity,
enchantment, attracts opposite sex

Marjoram joy, happiness, blushes

Marshmallow beneficence

Mint virtue

Moonwort forgetfulness

Morning Glory affectation

Mugwort happiness

Parsley festivity, joy, victory

Peppermint protection from
illness, warmth of feeling

Periwinkle love, sweet memories

Rocket rivalry

Rosemary remembrance, love

Sage wisdom, virtue, long life,
immortality

Spearmint warm feelings

St John's Wort animosity,
superstition

Sunflower adoration, loyalty,
haughtiness

Thyme courage, strength, elegance

Valerian cooperation

Vervain enchantment, superstition

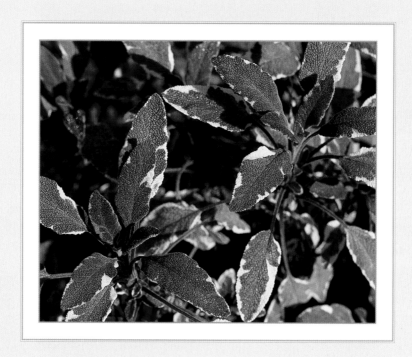

"Sage is of excellent use to help the memory, warming and quickening the senses."

NICHOLAS CULPEPER
THE ENGLISH PHYSICIAN ENLARGED
1653

Herb Glossary

BASIL *(Ocimum basilicum)*
Once an important medicinal herb, basil (*below*, also known as sweet basil) is now used mainly in cooking. It is a sun-loving, non-hardy annual plant that grows to about 90 cm (3 feet) high outdoors, but it is also very easy to grow indoors on a sunny kitchen windowsill. The closely related holy basil (*Ocimum sanctum*) is a sacred herb in India.

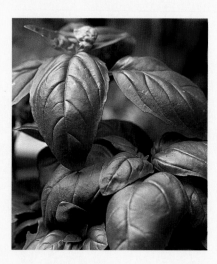

CLARY SAGE *(Salvia sclarea)*
This member of the sage family is a strongly scented shrub that grows to more than 90 cm (3 feet) high and wide. In herbal medicine it is used to treat stomach and kidney disorders, and in cooking it makes an interesting alternative to culinary sage.

COWSLIP *(Primula veris)*
With its crinkled leaves and bright yellow flowers, the cowslip is a familiar plant of the meadows and pastures of Britain, continental Europe, and Asia. Tea made with cowslip flowers makes a good nerve tonic, and cowslip roots are used in herbal cough remedies.

LAVENDER *(Lavandula officinalis)*
Lavender has long been treasured for its distinctive fragrance and powerful healing properties, and its oil is an essential ingredient in the perfume industry. Its purple, white, or blue flowers bloom in summer, and its foliage stays attractive all year round.

Madonna Lily *(Lilium candidum)*

Because its delicate white flowers were traditionally associated with purity, the early Christian church dedicated this plant to the Madonna (the Virgin Mary). A native of the Mediterranean countries, it was introduced into Britain in the sixteenth century and quickly became a favourite garden plant.

Marigold *(Calendula officinalis)*

The marigold, also known as the pot marigold, has pale green leaves and intensely golden-orange flowers. Its petals have antiseptic, antibacterial, and antifungal properties, making them very useful in herbal medicine, and they are also edible so they can be used to add a splash of colour to salads and soups.

Passionflower *(Passiflora spp)*

The many species of passionflower (*above*) are New World shrubs and climbing vines, some of which are now widely cultivated for their flowers and their sweet, juicy fruit. Passionflower extracts are popular ingredients of herbal remedies for insomnia and nervousness.

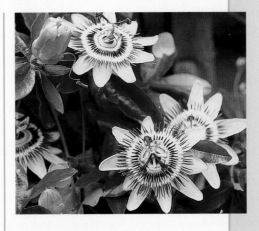

Peppermint *(Mentha x piperita)*

This hybrid of water mint (*Mentha aquatica*) and spearmint (*Mentha x spicata*) grows 30 to 60 cm (1 to 2 feet) high, but can reach 90 cm (3 feet) when in bloom, and is widely used as a medicinal and culinary herb. Its leaves contain a volatile oil rich in menthol, which is peppermint's main active ingredient and is mainly responsible for the herb's well-known flavour and its soothing and antibacterial properties.

ROSE *(Rosa spp)*
The countless modern varieties of rose
(*right*) are the result of centuries of
careful cultivation and breeding from the
wild species that grow across most of the
Northern Hemisphere. Their petals have
many cosmetic and medicinal uses and
provide an intensely scented oil for the
perfume industry, while their fruits (hips)
are a rich natural source of vitamin C.

ROSEMARY *(Rosmarinus officinalis)*
Originating in the sunny lands bordering
the Mediterranean Sea, rosemary (*below*)
has dark green, needle-like leaves with a
piney aroma, and its flowers range in

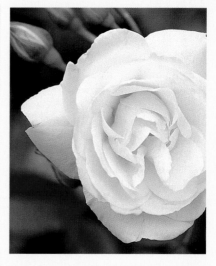

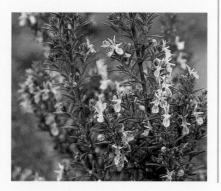

colour from white through pink to pale
blue or dark blue. It is a popular culinary
herb and a widely used ingredient of
herbal medicines and cosmetics.

SKULLCAP *(Scutellaria spp)*
The various species of skullcap grow
widely across the temperate regions of
the world, and get their name from the
distinctive shape of their seed capsules.
They have paired blue or pink flowers,

and their stems and serrated leaves are used in remedies for nervous disorders.

VALERIAN *(Valeriana officinalis)*
Valerian *(below)* is widely distributed throughout Europe and northern Asia, where it favours wet or marshy ground and the banks of rivers and ditches. It grows to a height of around 90 cm (3 feet), and its rhizome and roots are used medicinally as a mild sedative and to promote sound sleep.

VERVAIN *(Verbena officinalis)*
This slender, erect perennial, a common plant along roadsides, in meadows, and on waste ground, has white or lilac-coloured flowers and grows to a height of about 60 cm (2 feet). In herbal medicine, it is used both as a nerve tonic and as an antiseptic.

VETIVER *(Vetiveria zizanoides)*
Vetiver is a wild grass traditionally used in Asia for making mats, blinds, awnings, and thatched roofs. It is also used in herbal medicine to calm and soothe the mind – vetiver oil is known as "the oil of tranquillity" – and its earthy fragrance makes it a popular ingredient of perfumes and toiletries.

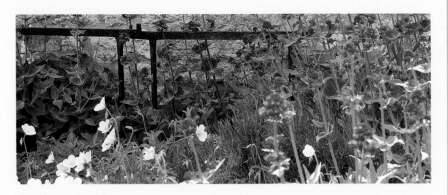

Buying Herbs

HERBS, BOTH DRIED AND FRESH, are now much more widely available than they were in the past. Most supermarkets stock a good variety of dried culinary herbs, such as sage, thyme, and basil, and some also sell a small range of the most popular fresh herbs including parsley and coriander. For the less-common herbs, and for herb oils, you will need to try specialist herb stores or Asian markets, or buy them online from one of the many websites that offer good-quality herbs and oils.

When you buy fresh herbs from a shop – loose in plastic boxes, in bundles fastened with rubber bands, or sometimes growing in small pots – avoid any that are limp or discoloured, or don't smell vibrantly fresh. Either use them straight away or dry them for later use, because they will soon start to wilt and become unusable, even if you keep them in the fridge.

THE HERBAL CABINET

When buying plants, make sure the leaves are whole, its stems are strong and both leaves and stems are evenly distributed. Straggly stems may indicate that the plant has not been grown in ideal conditions. If it's early in the growing season and the plants are displayed outdoors, check for brown scorch marks on the leaf tips, which may mean they have been damaged by wind or frost.

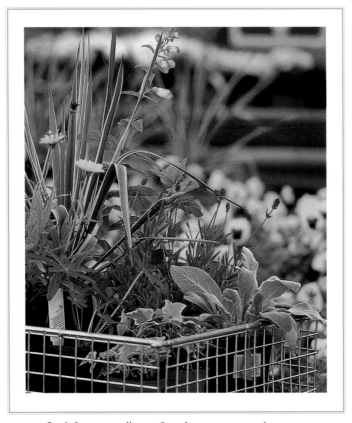

Look for strong, disease-free plants at your garden centre.

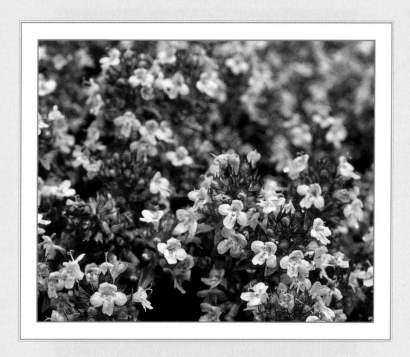

"Speak not, whisper not,
Here bloweth thyme and bergamot,
Softly on thee every hour
Secret herbs their species shower."

WALTER DE LA MARE
THE SUNKEN GARDEN
1917

Drying Herbs

BEFORE DRYING FRESH HERBS, first wipe off any soil but do not wash them, because damp herbs are more likely to become mouldy during the drying process. To dry them, first spread them out on clean, plain paper (not newspaper, because its ink can stain the leaves), or tie them into small, loose bunches. Then put them in a dry, well-ventilated room or cupboard where the temperature is around 24°C (75°F) – lower temperatures will increase the drying time, and at higher temperatures the volatile oils that give the herbs their flavour will start to evaporate away.

THE HERBAL CABINET

You can dry herbs in a microwave oven. Ovens vary in power, so experiment with the time you give each type. Spread herbs of a single kind on a paper towel and try 30 seconds on medium power and adjust accordingly. Aim to dry them thoroughly but not to the point of brittleness, as they may catch fire.

Depending on the thickness of the leaves, the herbs will take from one to four weeks to dry completely. When they are completely dried, gently strip off the leaves and put them in airtight jars. If you store the jars in a cool, dark, dry place, the herbs will retain their goodness for up to a year.

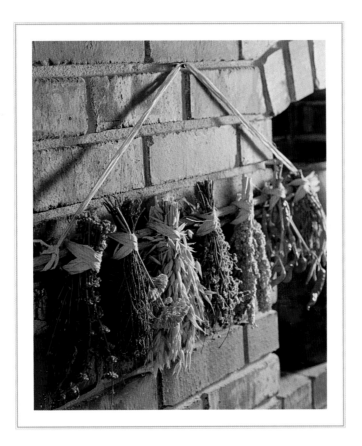

Freezing Herbs

FREEZING SPRIGS OF FRESH HERBS to preserve them is a quick and effective alternative to drying them, and it has the advantage of retaining most of their original flavour, and you can use frozen herbs in cooking in the same quantities as you would use for fresh herbs. To freeze your herbs, first wipe away any soil then divide the sprigs into small portions, each the equivalent of about 2 or 3 tablespoonfuls of leaves. Seal the portions into separate, labelled freezer bags, place the bags into rigid plastic boxes to protect them from crushing, and put them in the freezer.

THE HERBAL CABINET

Add frozen herbs to the dish you are preparing early on in the cooking so that their flavours can be fully absorbed. You don't have to defrost herbs before using them. It's a good idea to cover basil leaves with good-quality olive oil or melted butter before freezing them, as this layer helps them to retain their colour.

Alternatively, you can chop the herbs finely and put them into ice-cube trays, half-filling each compartment with herbs. Top the trays up with water, then freeze them. Once they are frozen, remove the cubes and put them into labelled freezer bags and store them in your freezer.

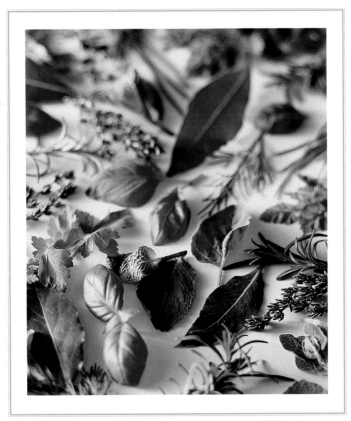

Freezing is a good method of storing herbs as both flavours
and colours are retained.

Index

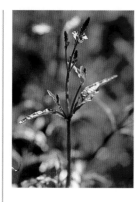